Alkaline Mediterranean Cookbook

47 Delicious Clean Food Recipes to Help You Enjoy a Healthy Lifestyle and Lose Weight without Feeling Deprived

By Elena Garcia

Copyright Elena Garcia © 2020

www.YourWellnessBooks.com

All rights reserved. No part of this publication may be reproduced, stored in a retrieval system, or transmitted, in any form or by any means, electronic, mechanical, photocopying, recording or otherwise, without the prior written permission of the author and the publishers.

The scanning, uploading, and distribution of this book via the Internet or via any other means without the permission of the author is illegal and punishable by law. Please purchase only authorized electronic editions, and do not participate in or encourage electronic piracy of copyrighted materials.

Disclaimer

A physician has not written the information in this book. It is advisable that you visit a qualified dietician so that you can obtain a highly personalized treatment for your case, especially if you want to lose weight effectively. This book is for informational and educational purposes only and is not intended for medical purposes. Please consult your physician before making any drastic changes to your diet.

All information in this book has been carefully researched and checked for factual accuracy. However, the author and publishers make no warranty, expressed or implied, that the information contained herein is appropriate for every individual, situation or purpose, and assume no responsibility for errors or omission. The reader assumes the risk, and full responsibility for all actions and the author will not be held liable for any loss or damage, whether consequential, incidental, and special or otherwise, that may result from the information presented in this publication.

The book is not intended to provide medical advice or to take the place of medical advice and treatment from your personal physician. Readers are advised to consult their own doctors or other qualified health professionals regarding the treatment of medical conditions. The author shall not be held liable or responsible for any misunderstanding or misuse of the information contained in this book. The information is not intended to diagnose, treat, or cure any disease.

If you suffer from any medical condition, are pregnant, lactating, or on medication, be sure to talk to your doctor before making any drastic changes in your diet and lifestyle.

Contents

Healthy Eating Made Exciting, Tasty and Fun! 9
What the Heck Is This Alkaline Thing All About? 14
The Oldest and Most Proven Clean Food Approach Ever Created
– the Mediterranean Diet 26
    Combining Alkaline with Mediterranean 28
Recipe Measurements 30
PART I 31
Vegetarian and Plant-Based Recipes 31
    Easy Vegetable Frittata Recipe 32
    Nutritious Eggs n' Asparagus 33
    Toast to the Greek Breakfast or Snack 35
    Greek Loaf Organic Bread Recipe 36
    Vitamize Yourself Up Mediterranean Fruit Salad 39
    Energizing Lentils n' Rice 41
    Nutritious Butternut Squash Salad 42
    Aromatic Avocado Toast 44
    Alkaline Vegan Mediterranean Bean Salad 46
    Home-Made Pita Bread 47
    Delicious Zucchini-Crust Veggie Pizza 48
    Hummus Extravaganza 50
    Easy Spicy Lentil Soup 52
    Aromatic Veggie Lasagne 54
    Catalan Dream Extravaganza 56
    Melanzane Mozarella Dream 58

- Kale Minestrone 60
- Italian Classic Pesto 62
- Qui-zpacho 63
- Alkaline-Mediterranean Basil-Tomato Bruschetta Topping .. 64
- Whole Wheat Pita Pockets 65
- Easy Spanish Aioli 66
- Almost Alkaline Greek Salad 67
- Greek Quinoa Salad 68
- Easy Italian Berry-Bean Salad 69
- Italian Style Farro Salad 70
- Nutty Aromatic Romesco Dip/Sauce 72
- Tzaziki Spread/Dip 74
- Delicious Greek Garlic Hummus 75
- Natural Banana Pudding 76

Part II 77

Recipes with Fish, Seafood and Meat 77

- Simple Spanish Tuna Salad 78
- Super Healthy Quinoa Pallea 80
- Mediterranean Tuna Burger 82
- Mediterranean Chicken Flavored Veggie Soup 84
- Catalan "Pan Tomaquet" 86
- Traditional Salmorejo 88
- Rosemary Chicken 90
- Whole Wheat Pita Pockets 91
- Delicious Greek Breakfast Pockets 93
- Greek Breakfast Shrimp on Toast 94
- Delicious Balance Fish Frittata 96
- Halibut on Tomato Toast with Salad 97

- Egg-Lemon Tuna Soup 99
- Arugula Tuna with Lemon Parsley Dressing 101
- Olive Green Veggie Salad 102
- Grilled Chicken Salad with Grapefruit and Avocado 104
- Simple Spicy Egg Scramble 106
- Turkey Broccoli Mix 108

Bonus – Alkaline Mediterranean Smoothie Recipes to Help You Look and Feel Amazing 109
- Cucumber Dream Creamy Cheesy Smoothie 110
- Cucumber Dream Creamy Plant Based Alkaline Smoothie ... 111
- Refreshing Radish Liver Lover Smoothie 112
- Cilantro Oriental Alkaline Keto Smoothie 113
- Vitamin C Alkaline Keto Power 114
- Hormone Rebalancer Natural Energy Smoothie 115

Free Complimentary eBook 116

More books by Elena Garcia & Your Wellness Books 118

Recommended Resources Mentioned in This Book 119

INTRODUCTION

Healthy Eating Made Exciting, Tasty and Fun!

Welcome to the World of Alkaline-Mediterranean Eating. A simple, hybrid diet approach aimed at enriching your diet with delicious and nutritious foods.

So that you can easily:

- Enjoy a healthy lifestyle without feeling deprived
- Make healthy eating exciting and fun and enjoy delicious, nourishing meals with your family and friends (no more "dieting"!)
- Combine nutrient-packed alkaline vegetables and greens with quality animal products, to create optimal balance (and never feel bored again!)
- Start losing weight naturally, simply by improving the quality of your calories and consuming delicious foods that can speed up your metabolism (without going hungry or feeling like you have to give up your favorite foods forever, and without the "yo-yo" effect
- Enjoy more variety in your diet and never again torture yourself with some fad or starvation diets
- Become an excellent, healthy cook and have everyone love you for it
- Enjoy more energy naturally, by giving your body exactly what it needs to thrive
- Feel confident and empowered knowing that you eat your way to vibrant health, while, potentially, reducing the risk

INTRODUCTION

of many preventable diseases, simply by eating more nutritious and delicious foods
- Gain more focus – so that you can perform better at work and feel amazing in your body

My goal is to make it as simple and doable as possible. So, we will be diving right into it! You can expect a simple-to-follow recipe and healthy eating guide!

Here's exactly what you will learn from this little book, as I guide you step-by-step on your journey to wellness through balanced eating:

Alkaline diet and foods deciphered – in this section, we will quickly have a look at the alkaline diet and foods. This section alone has the power to radically improve your health! You see, no matter what your nutritional preferences are, you can always enrich your diet with more alkaline foods like healthy vegetables and greens (even if you're not a vegetarian).

Mediterranean diet and foods made simple –then, I will guide you through one of the most delicious and healthy diets ever created – the Mediterranean diet. I will also show you a few simple tweaks you can make to your diet today to start enjoying the Mediterranean diet lifestyle!

INTRODUCTION

Finally, I will show you how you can combine the alkaline and Mediterranean diets so that you can create your own version of this hybrid diet.

The good news is that this new approach is very flexible. So, you don't need to stress out about complicated diets. You will quickly discover a few, easy-to-implement, flexible eating ideas based on the Alkaline and Mediterranean lifestyles.

For example – how to combine healing greens and vegetables with healthy protein and other superfood ingredients by creating mouth-watering dishes you will never get bored with! We are talking traditional Spanish dishes, such as paella, in a very healthy alkaline version, or delicious Greek-style salads you can make in 20 minutes or less (the more you practice, the quicker it gets).

***

Before we will get into the *Alkaline Mediterranean* hybrid diet, I would like to offer you free access to our *Wellness Lifestyle newsletter*.

When you sign up, you will receive free instant access to our book *Alkaline Paleo Superfoods for Optimal Nutrition*.

With *Alkaline Paleo Superfoods*, you will discover the best clean food combinations to help you create nutritious meals on a busy schedule.

You will also be receiving other valuable tips and recipes from me to help you stay on track so that you can create a healthy lifestyle you love.

INTRODUCTION

You can sign up on the next page and become a successful reader at no cost!

Wellness Newsletter & Bonus eBook

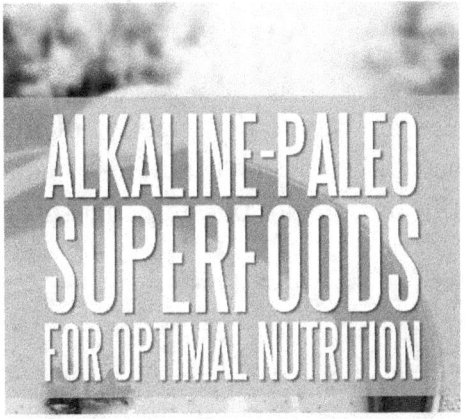

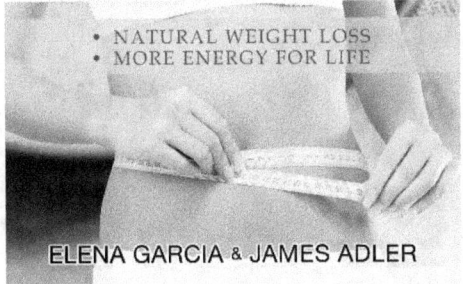

Sign up link:

www.yourwellnessbooks.com/newsletter

Problems with your download?

Contact us: elenajamesbooks@gmail.com

PART 1 – ALKALINE DIET & FOODS MADE SIMPLE

What the Heck Is This Alkaline Thing All About?

"Going green" is the way to describe an alkaline diet and lifestyle because the focus is on green vegetables in general, as they are the most alkaline foods you can possibly ingest.

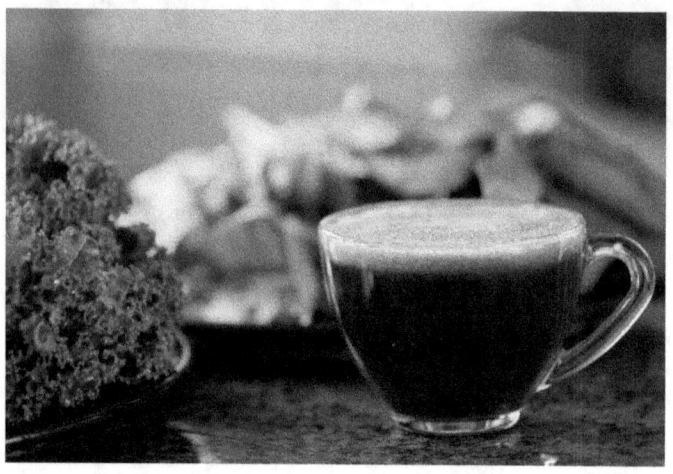

However, it's not about eating 100% green. That wouldn't be very doable!

It's all about adding more green, alkaline foods to your diet. This can be easily achieved by enriching your smoothies with leafy greens or adding a delicious salad to your meals. You can also add some leafy greens to your healthy (preferably made of low sugar ingredients) juices.

I have a couple of books dedicated to juices and smoothies (*Alkaline Ketogenic Juicing* & *Alkaline Ketogenic Smoothies*), in case you want to dive deeper into all kinds of healthy, healing concoctions. This book, will also show you different ways to help

you add more green, alkaline superfoods to your meals and drinks – almost on an autopilot!
There are multiple benefits of eating more alkaline:

Weight Loss
A diet rich in alkaline foods can assist you in losing weight. One way that it does this is obvious. The foods you will be eating are very healthy, rich in minerals, and low calorie in general.

Another benefit of an alkaline lifestyle regarding weight loss is that alkaline systems have more oxygen in their cells. Oxygen is a very essential part of eliminating fat cells from the body.

The more oxygen in your system, the more efficient your metabolism will be.

Natural Energy
Adding more greens into your diet does not only give you energy for the apparent reason that you are eating many more healthy, energizing vitamins. You are negating the acid-induced lethargy that is brought on by an unhealthy acid-forming diet (fast foods, sugar, processed carbohydrates etc.)

Not only do our bodies need an abundance of oxygen to lose weight, but we also need oxygen in our cells to energize us. The lack of oxygen in our cells causes fatigue. No, it is not just because you worked too late or partied to hard the night before. It is internal. If your cells are trying to function in a highly acidic environment, they will not be able to transfer oxygen efficiently; leading of course to exhaustion.

Cells in the body also make something that is called adenosine triphosphate (ATP). If your system is very acidic, it harms the ability of your cells to produce it. In the scientific world, it is known as the "energy currency of life." The ATP molecule contains the energy that we need to accomplish most things that we do (both internally and externally).

BODILY FUNCTIONS

Another benefit of the alkaline lifestyle is that your body will be able to function at an optimum level instead of being inhibited by acids:

- Your heartbeat is thrown off by acidic wastes in the body. The stomach suffers greatly from over-acidity.
- The liver's job is to get rid of acid toxins, but also to produce alkaline enzymes. By simply reducing your acid intake, you can internally boost your alkalinity thanks to your liver!
- Your pancreas thrives on alkalinity. Too much acid in your system throws off your pancreas. If you eat alkaline foods, your pancreas can regulate your blood sugars.
- Your kidneys also help to keep your body alkaline. When they are overwhelmed by an acidic diet, they cannot do their job
- The lymph fluids function most efficiently in an alkaline system. They remove acid waste. Acidic systems not only have a slower lymph flow causing acids to be stored; they can also cause acids to be reabsorbed through lymphatic ducts in your intestines that would typically be excreted.

MENTAL FOCUS

The alkalinity of the system is one of the best ways to focus and strengthen the mind. Just as the rest of the body is poorly affected by acid-forming foods and other toxins, so is your brain.

And as we all know, it should be possible to control your emotions and decision making with your mind. Guess what? If your body is too acidic and is not alkaline, your mental clarity will be cloudy, your decision making could be off, as well as your emotional state.

DETOX
Another huge benefit of an alkaline lifestyle is detoxification. First, you are going to be cutting out processed foods that are continually adding toxins to your system.

Secondly, you are going to be eating foods that allow your body to detox and rid itself of the acids that have built up in your system all this time. When we detoxify our bodies, our emotions, bodily functions, and mental functions can operate at their optimum levels.

Our bodies function optimally when our blood is at about 7.365 - 7.45 pH.

pH levels range from 0 to 14. 0 is the highest level of acidity, but basically, everything 0-7 would be considered acidic. The 7-14 range is alkaline.

Before we dive into complicated pH discussions, here is one thing to understand:
-The alkaline diet is not about changing or "raising" your pH. This is where many alkaline guides go wrong. You see, our body is smart enough to **self-regulate** our pH for us, no matter what we eat.

Unfortunately, when you constantly bombard your body with acid-forming foods (for example, processed foods, fast food, alcohol, sugar, and even too much meat), you torture your body with incredible stress. Why? Well, because it has to work harder to maintain that optimal pH...

Here's a simple example...

Imagine you immerse yourself in a bath filled with ice. You say, but hey, my body can self-regulate its optimal temperature, right? And yes, it can. But it will eventually collapse, and you will get ill. The same happens with nutrition and our blood pH.

You can spend years indulging in toxic, processed, acid-forming foods that only deprive your body of its vital nutrients, saying: "But hey, my body will self-regulate its optimal blood pH."

And again, it will...but sooner or later, it will give up and manifest a disease. It will accumulate fat as its natural defense function to protect your body from over-acidity. We don't wanna end up there, right?

Changing your diet to one that is full of alkaline foods is one of the easiest and best things you can do for your overall health. One of the easiest and most effective ways to do so is with salads. The good news is that you can say goodbye to boring, unappetizing, strictly alkaline salads make of broccoli, tomatoes, and cucumber.

We will be eating delicious and filling alkaline Mediterranean meals to get you closer to your health goals starting today!

Now, let's have a look at our alkaline food lists, so that you have a practical understanding of what alkaline foods and drinks look like.

I also recommend you go to our private website at:

www.YourWellnessBooks.com/charts
and grab your printable alkaline food charts to stick on your fridge or keep in your car, to have it ready when you go shopping.

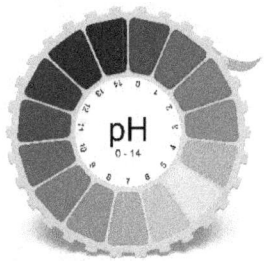

The recipes contained in this book are super rich in alkaline foods while taking advantage of traditional, Mediterranean clean-food recipes to help you create optimal balance and enjoy what you eat. If you don't enjoy it, it's hard to stick to it. That's my personal philosophy. Balance is key!

Ok, so now, let's have a look at our alkaline food lists:

Alkaline Veggies:
- Asparagus
- Broccoli
- Chilli
- Capsicum/Pepper
- Courgette/Zucchini
- Dandelion
- Cabbage

PART 1 – ALKALINE DIET & FOODS MADE SIMPLE

- Sweet Potato
- Mint
- Ginger
- Coriander
- Basil
- Brussels Sprouts
- Pumpkin
- Radish
- Snowpeas
- Green Beans
- String Beans
- Runner Beans
- Spinach
- Kale
- Cauliflower
- Carrot
- Beetroot
- Eggplant/Aubergine
- Garlic
- Onion
- Parsley
- Butternut etc.)
- Pumpkin
- Wakame
- Kelp
- Collards
- Chives
- Endive
- Chard
- Celery
- Cucumber
- Watercress

PART 1 – ALKALINE DIET & FOODS MADE SIMPLE

- Lettuce
- Peas
- Broad Beans
- New Potato

ALKALINE SPROUTS:
- Soy Sprouts
- Alfalfa Sprouts
- Amaranth Sprouts
- Broccoli Sprouts
- Fenugreek Sprouts
- Kamut Sprouts
- Mung Bean Sprouts
- Quinoa Sprouts
- Radish Sprouts
- Spelt Sprout

ALKALINE FRUITS:
- Avocado
- Tomato
- Lemon
- Lime
- Grapefruit
- Fresh Coconut
- Pomegranate

ALKALINE GRASSES:
- Wheatgrass
- Barley Grass
- Kamut Grass
- Dog Grass
- Shave Grass
- Oat Grass

ALKALINE NUTS AND SEEDS:
- Almonds
- Coconut
- Flax Seeds
- Pumpkin Seeds
- Sesame Seeds
- Sunflower Seeds

ALKALINE OILS:
- Avocado Oil
- Coconut Oil
- Flax Oil
- Udo's Oil
- Olive Oil

ALKALINE BREAD:
- Sprouted Bread
- Sprouted Wraps
- Gluten/Yeast
- Free Breads & Wraps

ALKALINE BEANS AND GRAINS
- Amaranth
- Buckwheat
- Chia/Salba
- Kamut
- Millet
- Quinoa
- Lentils
- Mung Beans
- Pinto Beans

- Red Beans
- Soy Beans
- White Beans

Go to:

www.YourWellnessBooks.com/charts

to download your printable PDF alkaline charts to help you enrich your diet with alkaline foods!

Does Going Alkaline Mean I Have to Eat ONLY 100% Alkaline Foods, All the Time?

No, luckily, it's much easier (and more flexible) than that. When it comes to the alkaline diet, there is something called the 70/30 rule meaning that about 70% of your diet should be fresh, nutrient-dense alkaline-forming foods and the remaining 30% can be acid-forming foods (however they still should be clean and organic, for example, grass-fed meat or organic eggs).

This is what we will be doing in this book! We will be creating, Alkaline-Mediterranean hybrid diet…So that we can combine greens and other alkaline foods with quality non-alkaline foods (such as seafood, fish or meat).

Imagine, some fresh salmon, served with a large avocado, lime juice, and spices.

Or…an amazing veggie salad with some tuna and organic cheese.

It's all about balance!

PART 1 – ALKALINE DIET & FOODS MADE SIMPLE

The reason I have been able to live an alkaline lifestyle for so many years now, is because I follow the 70/30 rule (sometimes 80/20). I love combining alkaline diet and foods with other healthy diets (paleo, keto or, in our case – Mediterranean diet).

That being said, once a year, I like to go on an alkaline cleanse and then, I detox my body by eating super alkaline foods! It helps me heal my body, get rid of stubborn fat and feel more focus and energy.

To learn more about my favorite alkaline cleanse, visit:

www.YourWellnessBooks.com/cleanse

I truly believe it can help you on your journey to vibrant health (and sustainable weight loss, if that is your goal)

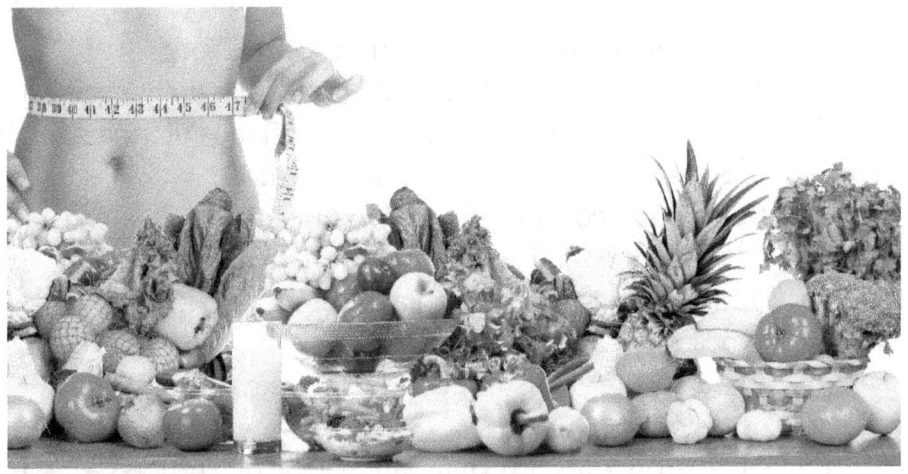

Now, let's have a look at the Mediterranean diet…

PART 1 – ALKALINE DIET & FOODS MADE SIMPLE

The Oldest and Most Proven Clean Food Approach Ever Created – the Mediterranean Diet

According to U.S. News & World Report the Mediterranean Diet is the best overall and easiest to follow.

It's still growing in popularity, with the latest research documenting its numerous benefits, and chefs and healthy food enthusiasts embracing Mediterranean ingredients and flavors.

It's basic run-down is this:

1. Consume natural, organic, unprocessed foods
2. Add more fruits and vegetables to your diet – serve your meals with fresh salads, and instead of snacking on processed sweets, snack on some fruit!
3. Reduce the consumption of red meat to once a week. Add fish, seafood, and occasional white meat.
4. Add good fats to your diet -avocadoes, organic olive oil, and avocado oil are very good for you.
5. Reduce the consumption of sweets only for special occasions
6. Choose organic, brown bread instead of a processed/ white.
7. You can include quality dairy products in small amounts. Personally, I like adding some quality goat cheese to my salads!
8. Add some nuts and seeds to your diet.

9. Legumes and lentils can also be turned into amazing Mediterranean dishes, as well! It's all about variety.
10. Make sure you drink enough water to stay hydrated, you can also make delicious smoothies (check out the recipes in the bonus section at the end of this book).

The Mediterranean Diet Benefits:
- Can prevent Parkinson's disease and Alzheimer's disease
- Reduces inflammation (it has an alkalizing effect on the body)
- Can prevent developing heart diseases
- Reduces risk of having stroke
- Improves mental and physical health and can even prevent depression and anxiety
- Is the best anti-ageing diet!

Combining Alkaline with Mediterranean

The basic rule to shift your meals towards an alkaline-Mediterranean friendly style is to:

- add more greens to your diet (can be done through salads, or you can juice the greens, or add them to your smoothies).

- add more good fats (for example fish, avocado, coconut oil)

Now, let's have a break from the theory and have a look at some delicious recipes to help you get started!

PART 1 – ALKALINE DIET & FOODS MADE SIMPLE

In case you haven't done so already, be sure to join our free wellness newsletter and get instant access to your free eBook: **Alkaline Paleo** superfoods.

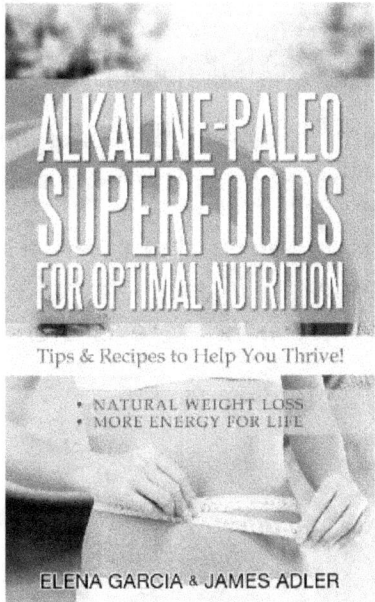

Sign up link:

www.yourwellnessbooks.com/newsletter

Problems with your download?

Contact us: elenajamesbooks@gmail.com

Recipe Measurements

I love keeping ingredient measurements as simple as possible- this is why I usually stick to tablespoons, teaspoons and cups.

The cup measurement I use is the American cup measurement. I also use it for dry ingredients. If you are new to it, let me help you:

If you don't have American Cup measures, just use a metric or imperial liquid measuring jug and fill your jug with your ingredient to the corresponding level. Here's how to go about it:

1 American Cup (1 c.)= 250ml= 8 fl.oz

For example:

If a recipe calls for 1 cup (1c.) of almonds, simply place your almonds into your measuring jug until it reaches the 250 ml/8oz mark.

I know that different countries use different measurements and I wanted to make things simple for you.

Recipes

PART I
Vegetarian and Plant-Based Recipes

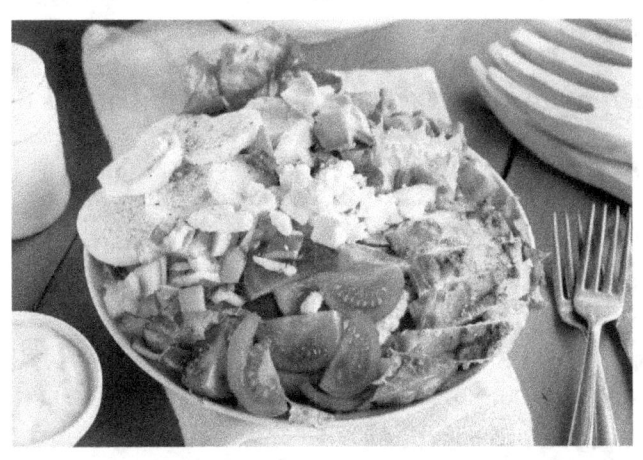

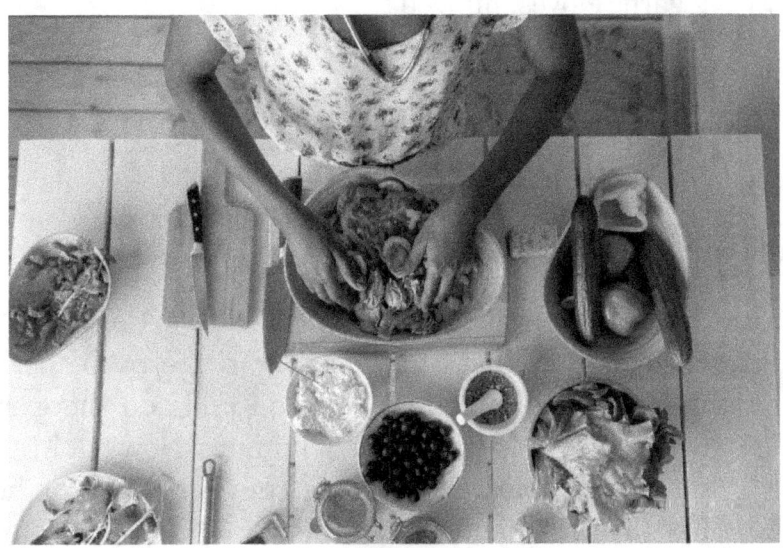

Easy Vegetable Frittata Recipe

This recipe is super quick to prepare. It makes a healthy and nutritious veggie meal! It is also super tasty and great for digestion.

This recipe can be served as a quick and nutritious dinner.

Serves: 2-3

Ingredients:

- 5 tbsp. olive oil (extra virgin)
- Total veggies=2 cups (use any amount of each: spinach, asparagus, kale, broccoli, mushrooms etc.)
- 1/2 red onion, diced
- 1 tbsp. parsley, chopped
- 2 garlic cloves, minced
- 6 large organic eggs
- 1/8 c. grated parmesan
- ½ tsp. black pepper
- Pinch of salt

Instructions:

1. Set your oven to 400 Fahrenheit (or 200 Celsius)
2. Using a pan that you can put in the oven, heat (over medium) the 1 tbsp. of olive oil and add the garlic and onion, brown for about three minutes. Now put in all of the other vegetables. Cook for 4-6 min depending on how you like them. Salt and pepper them.
3. In a separate bowl, whisk up the eggs with the cheese and pour them onto the veggies, so that they are covered evenly.
4. Now, put into the oven and bake for about ten min or until eggs are done. Enjoy!

Nutritious Eggs n' Asparagus

Asparagus and garlic have an alkalizing effect on this meal which makes it a perfectly balanced and healthy combination. The Alkaline-Mediterranean diet loves combining alkaline plant-based foods with quality animal products to create a perfect balance!

This recipe can be served as a quick breakfast, brunch or lunch.

Serves: 2-3

Ingredients:

- 6 organic eggs
- 30 trimmed asparagus, halved
- 1 1/2 cup sauce (recipe below)
- 1 tbsp. organic olive oil
- 1 clove garlic, minced
- 2 cups vegetable broth
- 1/4 cup Pecorino Romano, grated

Instructions:

1. Heat a large skillet to medium.
2. Add the olive oil and sauté your garlic. Let it brown, only cook for 2-3 minutes.
3. Stir in the sauce and broth with the garlic and blend them well.
4. Throw in your asparagus pieces, cover with a lid.
5. When the sauce begins to simmer, add the cheese and eggs.
6. Turn to low and simmer for ten minutes.
7. Enjoy!

Sauce:

- 2 cups canned plum tomatoes, drain, seed and cut into quarter inch strips
- 3 tbsp. evoo (extra virgin olive oil) 1 heaping tbsp. basil
- 1 tsp minced garlic cloves
- 1/8 tsp. salt
- 1/8 tsp. crushed red pepper

Sauce instructions:

Put everything into a medium sized skillet and heat to medium-high. Simmer for five min. or until most of the liquid is gone.

Toast to the Greek Breakfast or Snack

This is a delicious, healthy dessert or snack that takes only 5 minutes to prepare. I also like it for breakfast or after workouts.

It's tasty, naturally sweet and rich in protein.

Serves: 1

Ingredients:

- 2 Tablespoons of organic Greek yogurt, no added sugar
- 1 piece of organic toast (bread recipe below)
- 1 Tablespoon of raw honey
- 1 Tablespoon of pistachios (no shell)

Instructions:

1. Use the Greek yogurt as a spread.
2. Top with the honey and some pistachios!
3. Enjoy!

Greek Loaf Organic Bread Recipe

Nothing feels better than preparing your own bread. This process can be time-consuming so make sure you schedule it on your day off, or when you have more free time.

Ingredients:

- 1 ounce of fresh yeast or (2 tbsp. dry)
- 1/2 cup warm water
- Whole wheat flour (separate from the amount to follow) ½ cup
- 8 cups whole wheat flour
- 1 tbsp. salt
- 2.5 cup warm water
- 2 tbsp. milk
- 2 tbsp. olive oil (extra virgin)
- 1 ½ - 2 tbsp. raw honey

Instructions:

1. Dissolve your yeast in a bowl with the ½ c. warm water.
2. Add the half cup flour; do it slowly while mixing well.
3. Mix until it is not lumpy and is thick in consistency.
4. Set aside and allow it to rise for 15-20 min.
5. In a big mixing bowl, sift the other flour and salt, make a crater in the middle.
6. Put the honey, oil and yeast flour, and 2 cups water into it.
7. Slowly, pull the flour into the moist middle with your hands until it is well mixed, add more of the last half cup water if needed a little bit at a time.
8. Flour a working area and knead the dough until it does not stick to your hands.
9. Put your dough in a bowl that is lightly greased and roll it in the oil.

10. Cover your bowl with a dry towel, then a damp towel, and another dry towel over that one. Allow to sit and double in size for two hours.
11. Take out and place on a floured work area. Punch it and then knead the dough for five min. or so. Divide into three or four loaves. Shape into loaf of your liking and put onto ungreased baking sheets. Cover with 3 dishtowels as before and let them rise again for one hour.
12. Heat your oven to 425 Fahrenheit (or: 210 Celsius)
13. If you like, you can score the tops of the loaves 3 times for a crustier loaf. Place them right on the rack in the center of the oven for 35 minutes, or less if looking too browned. It should sound hollow if you tap it on the bottom.
14. Cool on racks and enjoy!

You can use it for sandwiches, toast, and bruschetta as well!

From Regular Yogurt to Greek Yogurt:

You can use yogurt tied up in cheesecloth setting in a draining bowl, or buy a yogurt strainer.

1. Line a mixing bowl with cheesecloth.
2. Put your yogurt into the middle.
3. Pull up the sides of the cloth and twist it so that the yogurt is completely encased.
4. Twist the top corners of the cloth in order to strain out the liquid over the sink. Do this until you get most of the moisture out.
5. When it begins to barely drip, tie it up tight.
6. Set in a colander over a bowl in your refrigerator for a few hours or overnight.
7. Place in the sink and press out any leftover moisture.
8. Open it up and scoop into a bowl. It should be thick like sour cream.

It also tastes great with nuts and berries! Find your favorite combinations!

Vitamize Yourself Up Mediterranean Fruit Salad

A natural fruit salad is a much better and healthier alternative to eating processed sweets and cakes.

It's easy to make and naturally energizing! I love it for breakfast or as a quick afternoon snack with some nut milk, or nut butter.

Serves: 2-3

Ingredients:

- One pint of strawberries
- A papaya
- ½ of a pineapple
- An orange
- A whole custard apple
- A mango
- A lemon
- 2 Tablespoons of raw honey

Instructions:

1. First, peel the mango, pineapple, and papaya. Chop them all up into one-inch pieces.
2. Put them in a large bowl.
3. Rinse your strawberries and take off the tops. Cut each into fours, then throw them in the bowl.
4. Squeeze both the orange and the lemon juice over the fruit, then add the honey and stir to blend all ingredients. Refrigerate for an hour or more.

Here is another version of this recipe, where you can add different fruits, just keep the quantities the same.

Ingredients:

- 2 cup pineapple chopped into one in. pieces
- 2 cup mango chopped into one in. pieces
- 2 cup papaya cut into strips
- 2 cup kiwi quarter and cut into half inch pieces
- 25 cherries, pitted and halved
- 2 cup peaches chopped into one in. pieces
- 1 cup peeled oranges seeded and sliced
- 1 cup peeled tangerines seeded and sliced
- 4 tbsp. fresh lime juice
- 4 tbsp. sugar
- 10 tbsp. water
- 1 pinch of salt
- 1 tbsp. lime zest

Instructions:

1.Mix up the water and sugar in a small pot and allow to come to a boil, make sure it dissolves. Stir and allow to thicken.

2Take the pan off of the heat and stir in zest; allow to cool.

3.Mix all of the fruit up in a big bowl and lightly salt. Add the lime sugar syrup. Toss the salad just a bit.

4.Cover the bowl and refrigerate for about two hours.

5.Serve with slotted spoon and enjoy!

Energizing Lentils n' Rice

This is a great, comforting meal for cold winters! It can be served for dinner, or even as a quick brunch.

Quinoa is a recommended alkaline grain as it's naturally gluten-free, rich in many nutrients and an excellent source of natural protein.

Serves: 2-4

Ingredients:

- 1 cup quinoa
- 1 cup green lentils
- ½ tsp Himalayan salt
- 4 cup water or veggie broth
- 2 large carrots
- Tahini if you like
- 1 teaspoon Italian spices blend

Instructions:

1. Go through the lentils and remove anything else that is in there.
2. Rinse them well under cold water. Get out a large to medium pot, put in the lentils and set on the stove.
3. Now, rinse the quinoa and add with your salt and water/broth.
4. Chop up your carrots and throw them in too.
5. Turn the heat up to high until the pot boils and then turn it down to lower setting. Keep it simmering, covered, for 45 min.
6. Add in the spices.
7. Turn off the stove and allow it to sit. Enjoy!

Nutritious Butternut Squash Salad

This delicious and nutritious recipe makes an excellent dinner and is just perfect for long, winter evenings.

Serves: 2-3

Ingredients:

- 3/4 cup quinoa
- 3-4 carrots (3 if large)
- Half cup lentils
- Half cup raisins
- 1 butternut squash (large ones are best for this recipe)
- 3 tbsp. extra virgin olive oil
- 2 tbsp. tahini
- 1 lime
- Pinch of salt/pepper
- Splash of apple cider vinegar
- 1 tbsp. rosemary (dried)

Instructions:

1. Preheat oven to 375 Fahrenheit (or 190 Celsius)
2. Take your squash and peel it, then slice in up into 1 in. pieces.
3. Put it on a baking tray. Drizzle over oil, along with salt and pepper to your liking. Cook for thirty minutes.
4. Cook quinoa and lentils together with water and ACV. Approximately 15 minutes.
5. Soak the raisins in a bowl of warm water.
6. Grate your carrots after peeling them.
7. Mix up the tahini, juice from the lime, and olive oil with a fork in a separate bowl.

8. Put everything into a large bowl, put the dressing on top. Toss well and enjoy!

Aromatic Avocado Toast

This outside the box, vegan-friendly toast makes an excellent breakfast – it's easy, nutritious and smells fantastic! It can also be used as a take-away lunch or brunch.

Serves: 1

First Variation:

Ingredients:

- Hummus (use store bought or one of the recipes in this book)
- Pesto (recipe in book)
- ¼ of a sliced cucumber
- ¼ cup sprouts
- 1 avocado (peeled, sliced, and pitted)
- Two slices of whole grain or wheat bread (you can use the Greek bread recipe if you like)

Instructions:

1. Toast two bread slices.
2. Spread the toast with some hummus.
3. Top with some pesto.
4. Lay cucumber on top of the pesto, add the sprouts, and then lay avocado on the very top of everything else.
5. Enjoy!!!!

Second Variation:

- Hummus (olive recipe)
- 8 sliced cherry tomatoes
- Pesto
- 1 avocado peeled, pitted, sliced
- Handful of sliced up baby spinach
- 2 pieces of toast (whole wheat/whole grain)

1. Toast the bread.
2. Spread the hummus and top with pesto
3. Place on the avocado, tomato, then the spinach.
4. Enjoy!

SO easy and yummy. You can add all different kinds of variations! Different spreads of hummus or pesto, different greens, and vegetables, even hot sauce or dressings!

Alkaline Vegan Mediterranean Bean Salad

Salad is a great way of accompanying all your meals to help you add in more nutrients so that you can look and feel amazing.

Serves:3

Ingredients:

- 1 can of cannellini beans, rinse and drain well
- 1 avocado, peel, pit and dice
- 1/2 cup yellow onion, dice
- 1 carrot, chop
- 1/2 cup spinach, slice thin
- ½ cup thinly sliced kale
- Splash of ACV (apple cider vinegar)
- Juice of one lemon
- 1 Tablespoon of fresh orange juice
- Pinch of orange zest
- 1 Tablespoon shelled hemp seeds
- ¼ teaspoon cayenne
- Salt/pepper to your liking
- A few Tablespoons fresh chives
- Some kind of toasted bread

Instructions:

1. In large bowl mash up beans and avocado with a fork.
2. When it is a nice creamy, chunky consistency it is ready.
3. Fold in all of the veggies.
4. Whisk up the juice and vinegar and fold this into the vegetable to combine well.
5. Allow to chill for one half hour.
6. Enjoy atop your toast!

Recipes

Home-Made Pita Bread

Enough to make 6 pitas. I like making them on Sundays to make sure I have fresh pita bread for my family for the whole week!

Ingredients:

- 2 cups water (warm)
- 4 tsp. instant yeast
- 1 tablespoon salt
- 4 cups flour (organic whole-wheat)

Instructions:

1. Mix water and yeast in a large bowl. Allow to set 5 minutes.
2. Slowly add salt and flour while stirring. Cover with a dishtowel and allow rising to occur for an hour.
3. Take out and put onto floured area. Knead it gently and re-cover for a half hour.
4. Set oven to 500 Fahrenheit (260 Celsius).
5. Split up the dough into 6 balls.
6. Roll out into eight-inch circles, as carefully as possible on one side.
7. Put the pita onto greased baking sheets and bake in the bottom half of your oven for 9 min. They should puff-up and be light brown.
8. You can cut them and open them or just use as bread! Enjoy!

Delicious Zucchini-Crust Veggie Pizza

This simple pizza recipe is yet another tasty way to help you add more veggies to your diet. Enjoy!

Serves:2

Ingredients:

- 4 cup fresh zucchini- grate and then chop - about 1 large or 3 very small zucchini
- 1/2 cup finely grated Mozzarella
- 5 tablespoons of almond meal
- 3 tablespoons fresh grated Parmesan
- 1 teaspoon oregano, dry Greek
- ½ teaspoon garlic powder
- ¼ teaspoon salt
- 1 egg, beat well
- 1/2 cup pesto sauce (recipe in book)
- 1-6 oz. jar artichokes, drain then chop
- 1/3 cup re-hydrated sun-dried tomatoes, slice
- ½ cup Kalamata olives, chop
- ½ cup spinach
- ¼ cup thin sliced red onion

Instructions:

1. Set oven to 450 Fahrenheit (or 240 Celsius).
2. Grate the zucchini with the large holes on a grater. Now chop it all up.
3. Put it in a bowl and put in the microwave for five minutes on high.
4. Line a strainer with a towel and allow it to drain until cool.

5. Squeeze the zucchini in the cloth to remove moisture. Then put it in a mixing bowl.
6. Mix in your cheeses, almond meal, garlic, oregano, salt and egg until well-combined.
7. Grease a cookie sheet with olive oil.
8. Divide crust in two and press it out by hand. Do not make it too thin.
9. Bake until it is firm and barely beginning to brown.
10. Turn oven down to 400 Fahrenheit (or 200 Celsius).
11. Top each crust with pesto and toppings and bake when oven is down to 400, just long enough for veggies to soften (5-10 min).
12. Serve right away and enjoy!

Hummus Extravaganza

Nothing tastes better than home-made hummus.

This recipe is enough to make about 2-3 cups of deliciously fresh hummus. You can serve it with veggies (carrots, cucumbers), rice dishes, or on a piece of toast.

Makes: 2.5 Cups

Ingredients:

- Fresh juice from two lemons
- One half cup water (from the cooking of the beans)
- 6 tablespoons Tahini
- 2 tablespoons extra virgin olive oil
- Two cups cooked garbanzo beans, soaked overnight and simmered a few hours, remove skins (optional) (save the water)
- 2/3 cup Kalamata olives, take out the pits
- 2-3 cloves of garlic, peel
- ½ teaspoon of salt
- Pinch of cayenne pepper

Instructions:

1. Mix the lemon with the water.
2. Using another bowl, whisk up the tahini and olive oil until they are smooth and well-blended.
3. Throw the garbanzos, cloves of garlic, olives and the cayenne pepper into your food processor or blender until they are smooth. Keep scraping the stuff off of the sides.
4. Keep the processor on and slowly add the lemon juice, mixed with the cooking water, for one min. Then keep scraping down the bowl.

5. Now do the same with the tahini and oil.
6. When it is smooth, put in a bowl and cover. Put in the fridge for an hour or so to let the flavors blend.
7. Enjoy with some home-made pitta bread (in moderation), or fresh veggies (in abundance!).

You can also eat this super delicious hummus on fresh veggies, sandwiches, wraps, salads, etc.

Easy Spicy Lentil Soup

Do you like spicy food? Try this amazing lentil soup. I recommend it for cold winter evenings. It has a nice, oriental touch that is energizing and refreshing!

Serves: 2-3

Ingredients:

- 3 tbsp. extra virgin olive oil
- 1 big red onion, chop
- 1 large carrot, chop
- 1 jalapeño, seed and chop up
- 1 1/4 cup lentils (brown) rinsed
- 2 leaves of bay
- 1 tsp oregano
- 2 tsp paprika
- 1/2 teaspoon ground cumin
- ¼ tsp of cayenne
- 1.5 cup tomatoes, diced (canned or fresh)
- 1 tbsp. tomato-paste
- 1 cup veggie broth
- 1 tsp salt
- 1 tsp fresh black pepper
- Chopped parsley (about a handful) red wine vinegar, and extra oil for serving.

Instructions:

1. Put the oil in a large pot and turn heat to medium. Put in the onion sauté for three minutes.
2. Next throw in the carrot and jalapeño. Cook, constantly stirring for three more minutes.

3. Put in your lentils, bay, spices, tomatoes/tomato paste, and the veggie broth. Turn up the heat and allow to boil, then turn to low. Put a lid on it. Allow it to simmer 45 minutes.
4. You may want to add more water.
5. Salt and pepper to your liking. Right before serving, add the parsley and a bit of the vinegar and oil.
6. Enjoy hot!

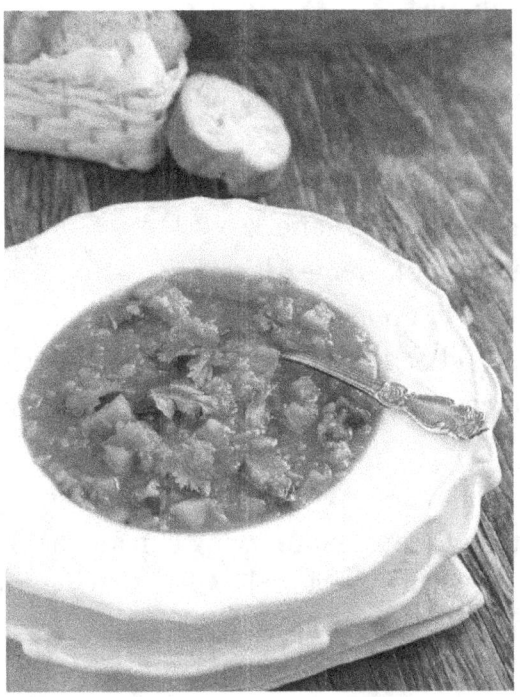

Aromatic Veggie Lasagne

This simple, and very aromatic veggie-style lasagne is designed to help you get hooked on veggies!

Serves: 4

Ingredients:

- 2 teaspoons olive oil
- 2 garlic cloves, mince
- 1 onion, dice
- 1 pound crimini mushrooms, slice
- 2-15 ounce cans of diced tomatoes (salt-free)
- ¼ teaspoon of salt
- 2 teaspoons of basil, dry
- 1 teaspoon of oregano, dry
- 1 teaspoon of thyme, dry
- Olive oil to grease
- 1.5 pound of eggplant, slice into thin circles
- 8 ounces of mozzarella sliced

Instructions:

1. Put the oil into a large frying pan and heat to medium-high.
2. Put the garlic in with the oil for two minutes, stirring the duration of that time.
3. Put in your onion, cooking another four min. Keep up the stirring.
4. Now put in the mushrooms and allow to cook for ten min.
5. Next, put in the salt, canned tomatoes, and herbs. Turn down the heat to medium. Put a lid on and simmer for about ten minutes. Make sure to stir a few times.
6. Uncover and stir for about 15 more min. Make sure you are stirring.

7. Set your oven to 325 Fahrenheit (or 160 Celsius).
8. Use a 9 x 13 pan and oil it.
9. Spread a layer, using half of the eggplant in the pan. Pour in half of your sauce.
10. Put in the rest of the eggplant as the next layer and then cover with the other half of the sauce.
11. Put foil on top and bake for a half of an hour.
12. Turn up the oven to 375 Fahrenheit (or 190 Celsius) and bake another half of an hour.
13. Take off the foil, lay cheese over the top and bake for ten more minutes.
14. Allow to set for 5 min and serve.
15. Enjoy!

Catalan Dream Extravaganza

This is a great family dessert that everyone will enjoy! It's naturally dairy-free, but still very creamy and delicious.

Serves: 4

Ingredients:

- 1 cup almond milk or rice milk
- 6 medium eggs yolks
- 1 cup of brown, organic sugar
- 2 tablespoons of starch or cornstarch
- 1 cinnamon stick
- The skin of half a lemon

Instructions:

1. Wash and brush the lemon peel. Peel avoiding the white part because it has a bitter taste.
2. Dilute cornstarch or starch in your chosen milk (about half a cup)
3. Pour the remaining milk in a saucepan and boil with the cinnamon stick and lemon peel. Remove from heat, cover and infuse warm to leave.
4. Meanwhile, whisk the egg yolks with sugar until white and mix with milk.
5. Add the cup of milk diluted with starch, mix well and let it cook on low heat, while still stirring until thick and creamy.
6. Remove the cream from heat ,take away the lemon peel and cinnamon and pour the cream into a wide source or small molds.
7. Cool the cream and set aside in the mold.
8. Put in the fridge and serve cold.

9. Serve with cinnamon and raw almonds if you wish. I also like adding a few raisins.

Melanzane Mozarella Dream

This dish requires rather long prep time- up to 2 and a half hours so make sure that you have someone to lend you a hand! Enjoy a nice conversation when cooking or treat yourself to a glass of organic wine.

Serves:4

Ingredients:

- 4 medium eggplants
- Half a kilo of ripe tomatoes
- 1 cup of fresh mozzarella cheese (check out in Italian food store to get the best one)
- 2 garlic cloves
- 2 tbsp. grated Parmesan cheese
- 3 sprigs of basil
- 4 tbsp. of virgin olive oil
- pepper
- sea salt or Himalayan salt

Instructions:

1. Wash the eggplant and dry it with a clean cloth and remove the stems from the tops.
2. Cut the eggplant, don't peel it, and slice it very thin.
3. Arrange the slices in a colander and sprinkle with salt. Let them drain for an hour to release the bitter juice out. Then, rinse quickly under running water and dry them carefully.
4. Peel and chop the garlic and tomatoes.
5. Cut the mozzarella into thin slices
6. Heat 2 tablespoons oil in a skillet over low heat and sauté the garlic.

7. Add the chopped tomato and basil. Add salt and pepper and sauté over medium heat for 10 minutes.
8. Finish the sauce by passing it through the food mill and set aside.
9. Stir fry the eggplant in batches adding more olive oil if necessary. Set aside when it gets brownish.
10. Finally, prepare for baking:
11. Arrange a layer of eggplant in the bottom of your baking dish and cover with a few tablespoons of tomato sauce and parmesan cheese.
12. Top with a cover of mozzarella (sliced). Then cover with tomato sprinkled with parmesan and bake for about 30-40 minutes in a preheated oven at 360 Fahrenheit (or 180 Celsius).
13. You can serve it warm or cold.
14. Enjoy!

Kale Minestrone

Who said that eating vegetables is boring? I can never get bored of this recipe. Feel free to experiment with your favorite spices to make this dish unique and to slightly transform it whenever you feel like!

Serves:4

Ingredients:

- 1 large red onion, chopped
- 3 carrots, diced
- 2 stalks of celery, diced
- 3-4 cloves of garlic, minced
- 3 potatoes, dice (1/2 in.) and rinsed
- 1 zucchini, sliced (half circles)
- 2 1/2 cups beans (cannellini), cooked or 2 cans, drain and rinse
- 1 can tomatoes, diced
- 1/2 cup quinoa or whole wheat pasta (uncooked)
- 2 cups kale, torn and tightly packed
- 7 cups boiling veggie broth
- 2 bay leaves
- 1 tablespoon oregano, dried
- ½ tablespoon dry thyme
- ½ tablespoon fresh rosemary
- ½ tsp cayenne pepper
- Salt/pepper to your liking

Instructions:

1. Get out a large soup pot and heat to medium high with two tablespoons of water in the bottom. The water will begin to boil, so you then need to put in onion, carrot, celery, and cloves of garlic. Allow them to cook for 7 minutes and stir often. You may need to put in extra water to keep veggies from sticking.
2. Boil the veggie broth in another pot and turn off heat.
3. In the first large soup pot, put in the potato, zucchini, tomatoes, bay, spices, and cannellini beans. Keep the temperature at medium high and keep stirring so that everything gets hot.
4. Put in the veggie stock. Put a lid on and let it boil. Then turn down and simmer for 15 min. (IF using quinoa add now)
5. If using pasta, add now along with the rosemary, allow to cook for five min.
6. Next, it is time to put in your kale along with salt and pepper to your liking. Stir and then allow the soup to sit, covered, for ten minutes before eating.
7. Enjoy!

Italian Classic Pesto

Pesto is delicious and naturally alkalizing. While it's traditionally eaten with pasta, you can also use it for your toasts, salads, quinoa, and veggies. You can also serve it with some spiralized carrots or zucchini. So yummy and healthy!

Ingredients:

- 2 cups fresh sweet basil leaves
- ½ cup extra virgin olive oil
- 3 tbsp. pine nuts
- Himalayan salt to taste
- Total amount of cheese needs to=¼ c. use Pecorino Romano and/or Parmigianino cheese.

Instructions:

1. Boil a pot of water with salt in it. While it is boiling, make a big ice bath in your sink.
2. When you see the water boiling, add your basil. Do this in several different batches. Leave each batch in the water for eight second and remove right away dunking straight into the ice water. Use a salad-spinner to drain or dry with paper towels.
3. Toast the nuts in a pan over medium heat until aromatic. Allow them to cool on a plate.
4. Crush your garlic cloves while the nuts cool and then blend all in the food processor.
5. Next put the blanched basil in with the pine nut and garlic blend. Process on high.
6. Slowly add the remaining oil and salt. Now add the cheese. Blend until it is a smooth as you like it to be.
7. Keep stored in containers in the fridge with a touch of olive oil.

Qui-zpacho

This is a combination of Spanish gazpacho and quinoa – the perfect recipe for a quick and nourishing meal.

Serves:4

Ingredients:

- ¾ of a bell pepper, de-seed
- ½ of a cucumber, peeled and sliced
- 2 ½ -3 cloves of garlic, chopped
- 1/4 cup of extra virgin olive oil
- 1 cup of cooked quinoa
- 6 tomatoes, peeled then quartered
- ½ tablespoon sea salt
- ½ tsp. red wine vinegar
- ¼ tsp. extra virgin olive oil

Instructions:

1. Put bell pepper in a blender. The garlic and cucumber are to be put in now as well. Only put 1/2 cup of the olive oil in there and blend until smooth.
2. Add quinoa, a little at a time, blending until smooth. Add tomato one at a time and keep blending until super smooth. Put into a bowl and add salt and cayenne. Cover and put in the fridge for 1 hour or more.
3. When serving, drizzle ¼ tsp. olive oil and some balsamic over each.

Alkaline-Mediterranean Basil-Tomato Bruschetta Topping

This is a simple, light dish that makes a perfect aperitif or a quick, refreshing, alkaline-rich snack.

People often ask me why tomatoes are considered alkaline-forming to the body. After all, aren't they acidic?

Well, yes, they taste acidic. However, they have an alkaline-forming effect on the body (it's because of the fact that they are very low in sugar and high in alkaline minerals, such as potassium). Exactly what your body needs to stay in optimal balance!

Ingredients:

- 1-1/2 lb. ripe tomatoes (about 5), cut into 1/4-inch pieces
- salt
- Pinch cayenne
- 1 clove garlic with a bit of oil mashed into a paste
- 2 leafy sprigs basil, chop roughly

Instructions:

1. Sprinkle salt over the tomatoes.
2. Drain them in a colander for ten minutes.
3. Put them in a bowl and lightly stir in the garlic, oil, and basil.
4. Sprinkle cayenne and fold in.
5. Enjoy! Goes well with a bottle of Sauvignon Blanc!

Recipes

Whole Wheat Pita Pockets

Whole wheat, home-made pita pockets can be a great addition to your vegetable soups and creams. Use them as a special treat!

Makes 8 servings

Ingredients:

- 3 ½ cup whole wheat flour
- 1 tbsp. active dry yeast
- ¼ cup water (warm)

Instructions:

1. Set oven to 500 degrees Fahrenheit (or 260 Celsius) and allow to preheat.
2. In a bowl, sift 2 cups of your flour with the yeast.
3. Once the dry ingredients are combined, mix in the water.
4. Add the other 1 ½ cups of flour slowly until the dough comes loose from the sides of the mixing bowl.
5. Now it is time to knead your dough. Knead well for four minutes.
6. Take out your dough and make it into eight evenly sized balls.
7. Flour a counter top or a large cutting board. Use a rolling pin and make each ball into a five or six in. circle. Do not roll them thinner than ¼ inch.
8. Spread some flour on each side of the pita.
9. Put each one on a non-stick cookie sheet and let them rise for a half hour.
10. Flip each one over carefully. Be sure not to pinch the edge or jostle them around too much.
11. Put them in the oven on the bottom rack and cook for five minutes, then remove.

Easy Spanish Aioli

This creamy-style dip is delicious, nutritious and healthy. It's traditionally served with seafood, however you can also use it as a bread spread or serve it with some veggies.

It also tastes delicious with fried potatoes!

Ingredients:

- 7 cloves of garlic, chop
- 1/2 tsp. salt
- 1 tsp. freshly squeezed lemon juice
- 2 eggs (yolks only)
- 2/3 cup olive oil
- 1 tablespoon fresh oregano, chop

Instructions:

1. Put your oregano, salt and the garlic into the processor and mix well.
2. Put in the lemon juice and egg, pulse again.
3. Slowly drizzle the oil into the food processor and pulse well.

Almost Alkaline Greek Salad

This salad combines balance, nutrition and taste. It always feels good to combine the healing benefits of alkaline veggies with super tasty Mediterranean ingredients.

Serves: 2

Ingredients:

- 1 pound chickpeas, soaked and cooked
- 5 tomatoes (big ones)
- 1 cucumber (large)
- 14 olives (Kalamata)
- 1 big red onion
- 1 bell pepper
- 1-4 oz. piece of feta cheese
- Some extra virgin olive oil
- Some dry oregano (Greek)
- Some red wine vinegar
- Pinch salt

Instructions:

1. Wedge tomatoes.
2. After peeling your cucumber, slice into half inch circles and half them.
3. Slice the onion up very thin.
4. Mix the tomato and cucumber together in a bowl. Add chickpeas and top with the onion and olives,
5. Now drizzle with oil and a bit of vinegar (2:1).
6. Add salt if you like.
7. Last step is to place a slice of feta on top and sprinkle the oregano.
8. Enjoy!

Greek Quinoa Salad

This is yet another delicious example of vegetarian-style alkaline-Mediterranean dishes. Quinoa is a miracle grain, it's super nutritious, rich in protein and a perfect ingredient for super healthy salads like this one. Pine nuts, mint and cheese give this salad an incredible taste!

Serves: 3-4

Ingredients:

- 1 1/2 cups quinoa
- 6 cups of kale, chop
- 1 red pepper, chopped
- ¼ c. pine nuts
- 4 oz. sphela cheese, crumbled
- 1 lemon
- 1/4 cup chopped mint
- 1 ½ cups red grapes, halved
- Extra virgin olive oil

Instructions:

1. To make the quinoa: Bring 1 1/2 cups of rinsed quinoa and three cups of water to a boil. Now turn to low, simmering covered for 15 minutes. Put the quinoa in a bowl in the refrigerator to cool.
2. In a bowl, marinate the kale with the lemon juice for a half hour.
3. Toss in all of the other ingredients (hold off on the oil).
4. When everything is well-tossed, you should drizzle the oil over the entire salad.
5. Enjoy!

Easy Italian Berry-Bean Salad

Berries are an excellent (but very often overlooked) salad ingredient and they taste delicious with some honey and balsamic vinegar.

Serves: 3-4

Ingredients:

- 1-16 oz. can green beans
- 1-16 oz. can chickpeas
- 1-16 oz. can kidney beans
- 1 whole bell pepper, slice
- 3 stalks of celery, chop
- 1 onion (green), chop
- 1 cup total berries of your choice, fresh or frozen
- 1/4 cup balsamic vinegar
- 3 tablespoons honey
- 1 lemon (juice from)
- 1 tbsp. extra virgin olive oil

Instructions:

1. Drain all of the beans and put into a big bowl. Mix in bell pepper, celery and the onion. Combine well.
2. In a blender or food processor blend berries, vinegar, honey, lemon, and olive oil.
3. Pour over the bean salad. Toss and allow to marinate for the night in the refrigerator.
4. Enjoy!

Italian Style Farro Salad

This recipe makes a very creative, nutritious and delicious dinner salad that is very likely to surprise all your guests!

Serves:4

Ingredients:

- 14 ounces farro
- 6 cups of vegetable stock
- 3 very ripe tomatoes, dice
- 12 leaves of basil (chopped)
- 4 garlic cloves, crush well
- 1/4 cup extra virgin olive oil (for cooking the vegetables, set aside 3 tbsp.)
- Salt and crushed red pepper to taste
- 1 large zucchini, slice
- 1 large red onion, dice
- 1 bell pepper, dice
- 1 eggplant (a smaller one)

Instructions:

1. Rinse the farro and remove anything bad in there.
2. Heat 3 tbsp. oil for cooking the veggies in the bottom of a pot to medium. Now add the garlic and farro. Sautee the garlic until it is golden brown, and toast the farro as well. Keep stirring so that it does not stick.
3. Now, add the veggie stock, a few spoonfuls at a time. Keep stirring while you are adding the broth, it will be evaporating. When farro is soft, it is done.
4. Heat up 4 tbsp. oil in another pan to medium. Mix the red onion, zucchini, pepper, eggplant, and tomato. Salt and

sauté until they are soft. If you run out of moisture in the pan, add a tad of veggie stock.
5. When the vegetables are done, take them off the stove and mix them in with the farro.
6. Add basil and crushed red pepper. Plate and drizzle with oil if you like.
7. Enjoy! A glass of Rosé? Yes please!

Nutty Aromatic Romesco Dip/Sauce

Romesco is a great dip for green veggies and is traditionally served with asparagus. So yummy and healthy!

Ingredients:

- 2 tomatoes ripe, oven roast
- 1 whole head of garlic, oven roast
- 2 dried mild chili peppers, rehydrate in water (do it overnight)
- 12 almonds, blanch (or purchase raw almonds without skin)
- 15 hazelnuts blanch
- 1 cup olive oil (extra-virgin)
- 1/3 cup vinegar (red wine or sherry)
- 1 red pepper (roasted and either in a can or jar), drain
- A tiny bit of cayenne
- A pinch of Spanish paprika
- Salt to your liking

Instructions:

1. First the chilies must be rehydrated. Do this by covering them in water for as little as four hrs. or leave them all night. When they rehydrate, take out the seeds.
2. Roast your tomatoes. Peel them and set aside.
3. Roast your head of garlic, remove from the shell and set aside.
4. Peel your almonds/hazelnuts. (add nuts to boiling water for one minute, take out and rinse them under cold water right away to get skin off easily)
5. Put all ingredients into food processor or blender and blend well after they cool to room temperature.

Recipes

6. Season with paprika, pepper and salt. Enjoy!

Tzaziki Spread/Dip

I love using this dip as a salad dressing (especially for salad with delicious olives and feta cheese!)

Ingredients:

- 3 garlic cloves
- 3 tbsp. fresh dill
- 1 cup cucumber
- 2 cups homemade/store bought Greek yogurt
- 1/2 tsp kosher salt
- 2 tbsp. fresh squeezed lemon juice
- 3 tbsp. olive oil

Instructions:

1. Throw everything into the blender or food processor and blend until creamy.
2. Put in the fridge for an hour or more.
3. Enjoy!

Use this versatile side as a sauce for baking, a dip for veggies and pita, or a spread! Both of these Greek sides would go well with a nice bottle of Athiri!

Delicious Greek Garlic Hummus

This super tasty and nutritious hummus can be used as a side dish, or a spread for your toasts. You can also enjoy it as a healthy snack, with some veggies!

Ingredients:

- 2 small garlic cloves
- 2.5 cup cooked chickpeas
- 1/2 cup tahini
- 1/2 tsp ground cumin
- 1/2 cup fresh lemon juice
- 3/4 tsp sea salt
- 3 tbsp. extra-virgin olive oil
- Dash of paprika
- A little extra olive oil to top

Instructions:

1. Allow chickpeas to soak overnight covered in water. They will double in size and loosen skins. Take off the skins, drain, add double the amount of water to more than cover and simmer for 1 ½ to two hours. Drain. Save the water.
2. Put the chickpeas into the food processor and pulse. Add tahini, lemon, and garlic, and pulse. Salt and cumin can be added now. Slowly add some of the cooked chickpea water and pulse until you reach desired consistency.
3. Put into a bowl, top with olive oil and paprika! So delicious!

Eat it on pita, whole grain crackers, fresh veggies, as a spread, or dilute 1:1 with water and stir with a fork to make a dressing! Other spices and roasted peppers can also be added. With hummus the options are pretty limitless.

Recipes

Natural Banana Pudding

This recipe is naturally gluten and dairy free and it doesn't need sugar...It's naturally sweet!

Serves:4

Ingredients:

- 5 ripe bananas
- cup of rice milk (to be boiled) , half cup of rice milk (not to be boiled)
- tablespoons cornstarch (eco)
- tablespoon of agar-agar flakes
- a few drops of lemon essence (suitable for cooking)
- 1 tablespoon of apple juice concentrate
- 1 pinch of sea salt

Instructions:

1. Boil a cup of rice milk with agar-agar flakes until dissolved.
2. Peel and cut the bananas and put them in the bowl of the mixer. Add half cup of rice milk and the remaining ingredients. Whisk and when it is a creamy, add the rice milk with agar-agar (dissolved).
3. Finally, put the mix in molds. Garnish with strawberries, blueberries or kiwis and a little bit of cinnamon
4. Let it cool down a bit and put in the fridge.

This is one of my favorite snacks and desserts for the summer!

Part II
Recipes with Fish, Seafood and Meat

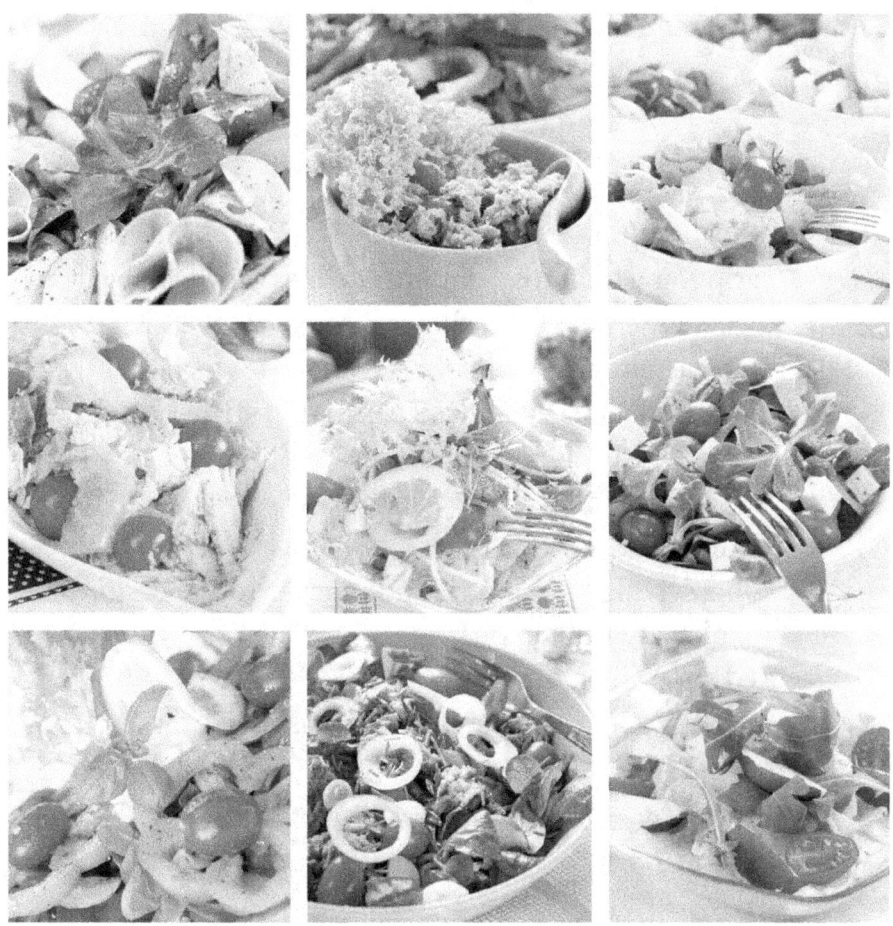

Simple Spanish Tuna Salad

This delicious recipe is low in carbs, abundant in clean protein, and high in nutrients. It's also very rich in good fats to help you stay full and energized for hours!

Serves: 3-4

Ingredients:

- 1 head of Romaine lettuce
- 2 rip roma tomatoes, cut into wedges (however big you like)
- 1 cucumber, peel and slice
- 1 can asparagus (white)
- 1 bell pepper, seed and slice into thin strips (lengthwise)
- 1 avocado, peeled, pit and slice
- ½ of a red onion, slice very thin
- 1 carrot, grate
- 2 hard-boiled eggs, peel and quarter (or trade for one can of albacore tuna in oil)
- red wine vinegar
- 2-4 tablespoons extra virgin Spanish olive oil
- salt (to your liking)
- 1 15 oz can artichoke hearts, drained

Instructions:

1. First, hard boil your two eggs. Then let them cool off in cold water and stick in freezer for a bit. When cool, peel and quarter.
2. Chop the whole romaine head in half and rinse and dry it.
3. Slice your tomatoes.
4. Slice cucumber after peeling.

5. Seed and the slice the peppers.
6. Grate carrot.
7. Open the cans of asparagus and artichokes and drain. Do the same if using tuna.
8. Tear up lettuce between two plates.
9. First lay on the tomato, then the cucumber, onion, pepper, and then carrots.
10. Break up the lettuce into small pieces for a salad. Make a bed of lettuce on a large platter. On top of the bed, place the tomatoes, cucumbers, onions, peppers and carrots. If using tuna spread it out around the lettuce.
11. Put the egg, asparagus, and artichoke on top.
12. Drizzle with oil and vinegar and salt to your liking.

Super Healthy Quinoa Pallea

This recipe is inspired by traditional Spanish paella, however, it uses quinoa instead of white rice, which makes this dish much more nutritious.

Serves: 2-4

Ingredients:

- 12-ounces of thawed shrimp (peel and devein)
- 2 carrots
- 2 turnips
- 12 asparagus, trimmed
- 2 young artichokes (make sure they are fresh)
- 1 lemon, cut in half
- 2 cup organic veggie broth
- ¼ cup extra virgin olive oil
- 2 cup scallions, slice very finely
- 2 garlic cloves, mince
- 1 ¼ cup quinoa
- 3 cup fresh peas
- 1 ¾ cup canned tomatoes (puree)
- ½ tsp of paprika (the sweet Spanish smoked variety is most authentic)
- Toast and pound ¼ tsp. saffron with a tad bit of salt.

Use a 13 ½ in. paella pan that you can put in the oven as well.

Instructions:

1. Rinse the carrots, turnips and asparagus and dry them.
2. Trim bottoms of the asparagus.
3. Trim artichoke as well.
4. Take the lemon halves and rub the artichokes with them. This will keep them from getting ugly. Put them aside in some lemon water.
5. Set your oven to 300.
6. Put the veggie broth in a separate pan and heat it up, but not to boiling.
7. Add evoo to the paella pan and turn the stove to medium. When hot, sauté turnips, asparagus spears, artichoke, carrot and onion for 2 min.
8. Put the garlic in the middle and cook for a few min. until all the veggies are soft and brown.
9. Now, put in the quinoa and continue sautéing until it turns clear. Do not let it get too brown.
10. Add your canned tomato puree and stir well. Add peas.
11. Let it thicken up and while scraping the pan at the bottom.
12. Next stir in the paprika and allow to cook for a couple more seconds.
13. Pour in the broth and add the shrimp. Mix it up very well. Allow it to boil. Now add the saffron and cook on high for about 15-17 min.
14. Put into the oven for 10-12 minutes.
15. Allow to set for 5 min and serve.
16. Enjoy! Goes great with a nice glass of Albariño.

Mediterranean Tuna Burger

This recipe is perfect for burger lovers! Why not enjoy a delicious burger in its healthier version?

You can even serve it with one of the salads from this book!

Total cooking and prep time for this recipe is about 1 hour (max), so be sure to try it when you have some more time to cook.

Serves: 4

Ingredients:

- 1 cup of fresh tuna
- 2 eggs
- clove garlic
- Some parsley
- Tomato
- Lettuce Hearts
- Turnips
- integral hamburger rolls
- Organic olive oil
- salt
- white pepper
- ketchup

Instructions:

1. Mash the tuna in a large bowl and add some minced garlic, chopped parsley, salt, pepper, and eggs. You can use a blender if you wish. Leave for about 30 minutes
2. In the meantime: peel, wash and cut the turnips into sticks.
3. Slice tomato and onion into rings.

4. Wash and slice the lettuce
5. Form the burgers from the tuna mixture. Fry.
6. Then, fry the turnip sticks in hot oil like potatoes.
7. Place the burgers on a hot plate with a drizzle of oil to make sure they remain juicy
8. Open the bread into two halves, add the burgers, sliced tomatoes and onions
9. Garnish with ketchup to taste.
10. Serve accompanied by fried turnips.

This recipe may even make you feel like you never want a traditional hamburger ever again!

Mediterranean Chicken Flavored Veggie Soup

This soup is simple, tasty, nourish and fun. It uses organic chicken broth (you can also make your own) and combined it with vegetables to help you create optimal balance. This delicious soup is great to enjoy in winter or when you are looking for natural recipes to help you fight colds.

Serves: 4

Ingredients:

- 4 cups organic chicken broth
- 3 medium sweet potatoes
- 2 medium zucchinis
- 2 leeks
- piece of celery with leaves
- cloves of garlic
- Lemon juice (from 1 lemon)
- 1 tbsp. of fresh mint
- 1 tbsp. brown, cane sugar
- Ground white pepper
- Salt

OPTIONAL: I like adding carrots and broccoli to my soups to make them super detoxifying. If you have carrots and broccoli, add them to your soup with the zucchinis (the last step)

Instructions:

1. Peel the potatoes, rinse and cut.
2. Wash zucchini and cut into slices, without peeling.
3. Remove the green leaves of leeks, cut into slices, wash and drain.
4. Prepare celery. Peel and chop the garlic cloves.

5. Bring the broth to a boil in a saucepan and add the potatoes, leeks, celery, garlic, salt and a pinch of ground white pepper.
6. Add the lemon juice and sugar and simmer the broth for about 20 minutes.
7. Add the zucchini and mint and cook for 15 minutes.
1. Serve the soup hot.

Catalan "Pan Tomaquet"

Would you like to discover my traditional, juicy bread? This is actually a typical Catalan way of preparing "tomato bread".

It is great as a snack or aperitif. You can also serve it with salads and seafood.

Super quick prep time only 10 minutes

Serves: 4

Ingredients:

- loaf of gluten free, organic bread of your choice
- ripe tomatoes
- anchovies in brine
- Extra virgin olive oil
- Marine salt

Instructions:

1. Cut bread in small slices
2. Cut the tomatoes in halves; use them to run inside the bread so that it absorbs the juice and pulp of the tomato until completely red.
3. Smear the bread with a little bit of olive oil (not too much as the anchovies are already oily and salty)
4. Add the anchovies and enjoy!

OPTIONAL:

Apart from tomatoes, you can also use some garlic and rub it on your bread. It gives it a really nice taste! I also love adding some fresh rosemary! I love serving pan tomaquet with some tuna and sardines.

Traditional Salmorejo

This recipe is very similar to Spanish gazpacho but is a bit more complex. It is a really refreshing and energy providing dish, perfect for hot summers.

Serves:2

Ingredients:

- 6 large ripe tomatoes
- cloves of garlic
- 1 egg yolk (cooked)
- thick slice of organic bread
- Olive oil (about 2-3 tablespoons)
- tbsp. white wine vinegar
- Water
- Salt
- Half cup of organic ham (it can be also chicken or even seafood. I have also tried replacing meat with tofu, it's up to you which option you choose)
- boiled egg
- 1 small onion
- 1 green pepper

Instructions:

1. Peel the tomatoes and cut them.
2. Peel the garlic and cut into small pieces.
3. Moisten the bread with water.
4. Add: Garlic, egg yolk, tomatoes, olive oil and bread crumbs to a blender or a food processor.
5. Season with some salt and vinegar (about 2 tablespoons). Set aside to cool down in a fridge.

6. On a separate dish, prepare cut hum pieces, chopped hard-boiled eggs, and the rest of the ingredients you would like to see in your soup. Use your imagination.

Unlike gazpacho, this soup is supposed to be dense and thick. It is traditionally served with ham, but you can experiment by adding some veggies, seafood or nuts. I usually check what I have left in my kitchen and do my salmorejo recycling!

Rosemary Chicken

This can be a nice family meal so make sure that everyone is involved in cooking! Rosemary chicken is just a classic in Spanish cuisine. Rosemary is actually the most popular herb used in Spanish cooking and was even dubbed "the queen of all herbs".

Serves:4

Ingredients:

- chicken 1.5 Kg (3.3 lb)
- lemon
- sprig of fresh rosemary
- half cup dry white wine
- 1 tbsp. olive oil
- pepper

Instructions:

1. Clean chicken. Wash and dry it.
2. Wash the lemon, dry it and insert it inside the chicken.
3. Arrange the chicken in a baking dish with 2 tablespoons of olive oil. Sprinkle with chopped rosemary, put it in a preheated oven at 360 Fahrenheit (or 180 Celsius) and bake for 1 hour and 10 minutes. Turn over halfway through cooking.
4. Remove chicken from oven and retrieve the cooking juices (we will need it for the sauce).
5. Heat the wine in a saucepan and simmer for 2 minutes to reduce slightly. Then add the cooking juices and remove the sauce from heat.
6. Serve chicken with this natural sauce.

Recipes

Whole Wheat Pita Pockets

Whole wheat, home-made pita pockets can be a great addition to your vegetable soups and creams. Use them as a special treat!

Makes 8 servings

Ingredients:

- 3 ½ cup whole wheat flour
- 1 tbsp. active dry yeast
- ¼ cup water (warm)

Instructions:

12. Set oven to 500 degrees Fahrenheit (or 260 Celsius) and allow to preheat.
13. In a bowl, sift 2 cups of your flour with the yeast.
14. Once the dry ingredients are combined, mix in the water.
15. Add the other 1 ½ cups of flour slowly until the dough comes loose from the sides of the mixing bowl.
16. Now it is time to knead your dough. Knead well for four minutes.
17. Take out your dough and make it into eight evenly sized balls.
18. Flour a counter top or a large cutting board. Use a rolling pin and make each ball into a five or six in. circle. Do not roll them thinner than ¼ inch.
19. Spread some flour on each side of the pita.
20. Put each one on a non-stick cookie sheet and let them rise for a half hour.
21. Flip each one over carefully. Be sure not to pinch the edge or jostle them around too much.
22. Put them in the oven on the bottom rack and cook for five minutes, then remove.

23. After they are cool, place them in freezer zip-locks. Remove before using. They defrost very quickly!
24. When ready to use, slice them in half and fill! They can be re-warmed for a couple minutes in your oven at 350 degrees.

Tip: When you are allowing the pita to rise, place them on cheesecloth or a thin kitchen towel, and cover with another towel. Turn them before baking by removing the top towel and using the bottom towel to flip the pita dough.

Delicious Greek Breakfast Pockets

This delicious recipe makes a perfect breakfast if you wake up hungry. It balances animal products with energy-boosting greens, like spinach.

Serves 2

Ingredients:

- 2 whole wheat pita pockets (home-made or bought)
- 6 egg whites
- 1/4 lb. turkey sausage (ground, 6 cut up links, or 3-4 patties)
- ½ tsp. chopped dill
- 1-2 cups spinach
- ½ tsp. each salt and pepper
- Greek yogurt (a dollop or two-recipe above) * optional

Instructions:

1. Cook the sausage in a frying pan according to directions.
2. Crack eggs, separate egg whites into a bowl, season, and whisk.
3. Add eggs to the cooked sausage in the same pan (draining grease first if you like) and cook over medium, stirring regularly for 3-5 min.
4. When eggs are almost done add spinach and dill. Allow it to slightly wilt and turn off the heat.
5. Add egg/sausage mixture to the pita pockets and throw in a dollop of Greek yogurt.
6. Serve with some fresh spinach!
7. Enjoy!

Greek Breakfast Shrimp on Toast

I am no a big meat person, but I love seafood! Also, usually, I just have a quick smoothie for breakfast. However, I love this recipe for special and family occasions.

Serves 4

Ingredients:

- 1/3 cup olive oil
- lb. shrimp (peel and de-vein)
- minced garlic cloves
- tomatoes (seed and chop)
- ½ bunch chopped green onion
- ½ c. feta (crumble)
- ½ of a lemon squeezed
- 1 tbsp. dry oregano
- 1 tsp dry thyme
- 1 tsp dry basil
- 1 tsp dry marjoram
- 1 tsp each dry onion and garlic (minced)
- Mix and store in airtight container.
- Greek loaf sliced (recipe above) into ½ in. slices

Instructions:

1. Place a large frying pan on the stove with 1 tablespoon oil and heat to medium high.
2. Add shrimp and garlic, sautéing for 4 min.
3. Remove from heat, place in a bowl, and chill.
4. Mix the tomatoes, 1 tablespoon olive oil, Greek seasoning, lemon juice, feta, and onion in another bowl and chill.

5. Take your bread slices and place them on a cookie sheet, brushing each one with olive oil. Place them in an oven set to 375 degrees Fahrenheit (or 190 Celsius) for 7-8 min.
6. When the bread is toasted, place some shrimp on each slice and top with tomato/cheese mixture.
7. Enjoy!

Delicious Balance Fish Frittata

This delicious recipe is also paleo and keto friendly. It fuses the revitalizing power of vegetables with quality animal products to help you create optimal balance.

Serves 4

Ingredients:

- 8 free-range eggs
- 1 teaspoon pepper
- 1 teaspoon crushed red pepper
- Half teaspoon salt
- Any other seasonings of your choice
- 1 cup canned salmon
- ½ cup chopped bell pepper
- ½ cup chopped spinach
- ½ cup chopped kale

Instructions:

1. Set your oven to 350 degrees Fahrenheit (or 175 Celsius)
2. Grease a 9 in. pie or cake pan.
3. In a bowl, whisk eggs, peppers, salt, and any other seasoning.
4. Place salmon and veggies in the bottom of your pan.
5. Now, carefully pour your eggs and seasonings over the fish and veggies.
6. Place the pan onto the middle rack in the oven for about 35 min. or until it is golden and firm.
7. Enjoy!

Halibut on Tomato Toast with Salad

This tasty recipe makes an excellent weekend dinner and goes really well with a big bowl of fresh salad.

Serves 6

Ingredients:

Toast

- 6 slices of thick crusty whole grain bread
- 4 cloves of garlic cut in half
- 3 ripe tomatoes cut in half
- Extra virgin olive oil
- Sea salt

Halibut

- ¼ c. fresh squeezed lemon juice
- ¼ cup extra virgin olive oil
- 4 cloves garlic (mince)
- 2 tablespoons paprika
- 2 tablespoons cumin
- 1 teaspoon salt
- ¼ tsp pepper
- 1 lbs. halibut filets (skinless)
- lemon (cut into 6 wedges)

Instructions:

1. In a mixing bowl, mix lemon, olive oil, minced garlic, paprika, half the salt and half the pepper.
2. Place fish in a baking dish. Marinate by rubbing marinade into both sides of the filets and allow to sit in fridge overnight.
3. Heat a grill or broiler. Season halibut with the rest of the salt and pepper. Cook for 3 minutes on each side.
4. Prepare toast.
5. Slice the bread and toast it.
6. Rub one side of toast with garlic.
7. Next, rub with tomato, while pushing down and squeezing in order to get pulp all over the toast.
8. Put one piece of toast on each place and top with halibut. Serve with lemon wedge. Serve sauce separately if desired.
9. Enjoy!

Egg-Lemon Tuna Soup

This recipe is original, tasty, nutritious and delicious. Tuna can make an amazing soup!

Serves 5-6

Ingredients:

- 3 carrots (chopped)
- 2 brown onions (chopped)
- 3-5 oz. cans tuna in oil (drained)
- 3 tablespoons fresh squeezed lemon juice
- ½ cup brown rice
- 5 cups vegetable broth (stock)
- 1 cup water
- 1 tbsp extra virgin olive oil
- Himalayan salt to taste
- 3 organic eggs

Instructions:

1. Cook brown rice according to the package.
2. While that is cooking, put a medium sized pot on the stove and heat oil to medium-high. Add onion and sauté for 5 minutes.
3. Add the veggie broth and the water to the cooked onions and simmer.
4. When the rice is finished, add the it to the onion broth, along with the drained tuna. Allow to simmer for 7 minutes.
5. In a separate bowl, whisk the eggs well. Add the lemon juice while continuing to whisk. Keep whisking until well blended.
6. Next, ladle in one full scoop of broth, still whisking constantly with the other hand. Repeat one more time.

7. Take the soup pot off of the heat and whisk as you add the egg/broth into the pot.
8. Enjoy!

Arugula Tuna with Lemon Parsley Dressing

This salad offers an incredible mix of clean protein, good fats, and superfood greens. The alkaline keto way!

Serves: 2
Ingredients
For the Salad:
- 1 whole scallion, finely chopped
- 2 cups of fresh arugula, chopped
- 1 avocado, peeled, pitted and sliced
- Fresh chopped parsley for topping
- 2 cans of organic tuna in olive oil

For the dressing:
- 4 tablespoons of thick coconut milk
- 4 tablespoons of parsley, chopped
- 2 tablespoons organic lemon juice
- 2 pinches of Himalayan salt (you can always add more if you need to)
- A pinch of black pepper and chili (optional)
- 1 big garlic clove, peeled

Instructions:
1. Combine all the salad ingredients in a big salad bowl and toss well.
2. Mix all the salad dressing ingredients using a small hand blender,
3. Pour the dressing over the salad and stir well.
5. Serve and enjoy!

Olive Green Veggie Salad

This salad is an excellent solution if you are looking for a meal replacing salad, something that will keep you full for many hours. It's a great mix of veggies, protein, and healthy, alkaline-keto fats!

Serves: 2
Ingredients
For the Salad:
- A few tablespoons of green olives
- 1 cucumber, peeled and finely chopped
- A few onion rings
- A handful of fresh baby spinach leaves
- 1 big garlic clove, peeled
- Half cup black olives pitted
- A few tomato slices
- A few almonds
- 2 cans of organic tuna

For dressing:
- 2 tablespoons of organic Dijon mustard
- 2 tablespoons of organic olive oil
- A few fresh basil and parsley leaves (optional)
- 1 tablespoon of coconut vinegar
- Black pepper to taste

Instructions:

1. Combine all the salad ingredients in a big salad bowl and toss well.
2. Mix all the salad dressing ingredients. You can use a small hand blender, or quickly combine and stir all the ingredients in a small bowl.
3. Pour the dressing over the salad and toss well.
4. Sprinkle over a few mint, parsley, and cilantro leaves.
5. Serve and enjoy!

Grilled Chicken Salad with Grapefruit and Avocado

This keto-friendly dish is served with delicious alkaline fruits. It's perfect as a quick, comforting dinner recipe.

Serves: 2-3
Ingredients
For the Salad:
- 4 skinless chicken breast halves (remove the bones)
- 8 cups of mixed salad greens
- 1 cup of grapefruit chunks
- 3/4th cup of avocado, peeled and diced
- 3/4th teaspoon of grated fresh ginger

For the Dressing:
- 2 tablespoons of low carb mango chutney
- 2 tablespoons of olive oil
- 2 tablespoons of fresh lime juice
- 1 tablespoon of coconut aminos
- Cooking spray

Instructions:
1. Preheat a grill and grease it with some cooking spray.
2. Take a bowl and combine the coconut aminos, chutney, lime juice, olive oil, and ginger in it. Keep aside.
3. Lay the chicken breast halves on a flat surface and brush those with 2 tablespoons of the chutney mixture.
4. Grill the chicken for 4 minutes on each side while coating lightly with the chutney mixture again on flipping. Remove from grill once done.

5. Cut the chicken into diagonal pieces. Lay the avocado slices, grapefruit, and salad greens on the plate and place the chicken pieces on top to serve. Enjoy!

Simple Spicy Egg Scramble

This recipe is perfect as a tasty, energizing breakfast or a quick meal.

Feel free to experiment with all kinds of spices for this one. Personally, I love chili powder!

Servings: 1-2

Ingredients:

- 2 tablespoons coconut oil
- Half cup shredded chicken
- 6 eggs
- 2 tablespoons coconut cream or thick coconut milk
- Pinch of chili powder
- Pinch of Pink Himalayan salt
- Pinch of freshly ground black pepper
- ½ cup shredded cheese
- Half cup green bell pepper, sliced
- A handful of chopped chive and dill

Instructions:

1. In a large skillet over medium-high heat, melt the coconut oil.
2. Add the chicken and sauté for 5 minutes until cooked.
3. In a separate bowl, whisk the eggs until frothy.
4. Now add the cream, salt, and spices.
5. Whisk to blend thoroughly.
6. Add the egg mixture to skillet with chicken and heat (on low heat) until almost cooked through, about 4 minutes.

7. When the eggs are almost done, add in shredded cheese and bell pepper.
8. Serve hot with some fresh chives and dill.

Turkey Broccoli Mix

This recipe proves how delicious and healing the alkaline keto mix can be.

Good fats, lean protein, and green veggies really help your body thrive and transform on a deeper level.

Servings: 2-3

- 6 turkey slices (thin)
- 1 small broccoli, cut into small florets, steamed or lightly cooked
- 4 garlic cloves, minced
- 1 small onion, diced
- 4 large eggs
- 2 tablespoon olive oil,
- Pink Himalayan salt
- Freshly ground black pepper

Instructions:

1. In a large skillet over medium-high heat, stir-fry the turkey slices in coconut oil (for about 2)

2. Turn the heat down to medium, and add the steamed broccoli florets, garlic, and onion.

3. Sautee for a few minutes.

4. When the veggies get tender, add the eggs by scrambling them all over the skillet. Keep stir frying until the eggs are set.

5. Sprinkle the olive oil on top, and serve hot.

Bonus – Alkaline Mediterranean Smoothie Recipes to Help You Look and Feel Amazing

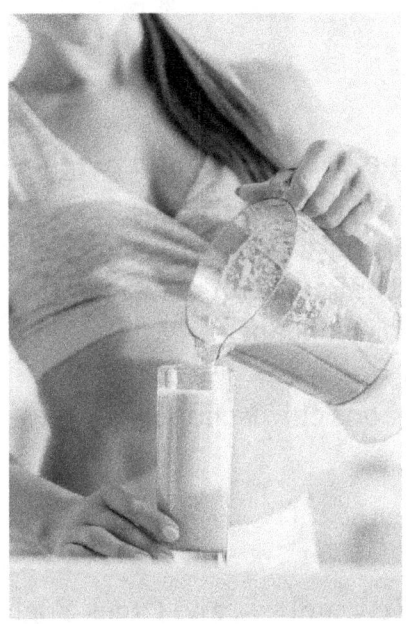

The following smoothie recipes are perfect if you are pressed for time. Some can be even served as a tasty and satisfying meal replacement!

Bonus – Mediterranean Smoothie Recipes

Cucumber Dream Creamy Cheesy Smoothie

This is one of my favorite "on the go" smoothie recipes as it doesn't require that many ingredients.

It can also be transformed into a delicious raw soup.

I have created a fully plant-based version of this recipe which you can check out on the next page.

Servings: 2-3

Ingredients:

- 2 big cucumbers, peeled and roughly sliced
- 1 cup full-fat Greek Yoghurt
- 4 tablespoons grated goat cheese
- Pinch of Himalaya salt to taste
- Pinch of black pepper to taste
- 6 radishes, sliced
- 2 tablespoons chive, chopped

Instructions:

1. Place the cucumbers, and Greek Yoghurt in a blender.
2. Add the Himalaya salt and black pepper.
3. Blend well and pour into a smoothie glass or a small soup bowl.
4. Add in the radishes and chive.
5. Mix well and add more Himalaya salt and black pepper if needed.
6. Sprinkle the cheese and enjoy!

Cucumber Dream Creamy Plant Based Alkaline Smoothie

This is a plant-based version of the previous recipe. It also tastes delicious, and I highly recommend it for days where your goal is detoxification to have more energy.

Servings: 2-3

Ingredients:

- 2 big cucumbers, peeled and roughly sliced
- 1 big avocado
- 1 cup of coconut milk
- 1 small lemon, peeled and sliced
- 4 tablespoons cashews, chopped or powdered
- Pinch of Himalaya salt to taste
- Pinch of black pepper to taste
- 6 radishes, sliced
- 2 tablespoons chive, chopped

Instructions:

1. Place the cucumbers, coconut milk, avocado and lemon in a blender.
2. Add the Himalaya salt and black pepper.
3. Blend well and pour into a smoothie glass or a small soup bowl.
4. Add in the radishes and chive.
5. Mix well and add more Himalaya salt and black pepper if needed.
6. Sprinkle the cashews and enjoy!

Refreshing Radish Liver Lover Smoothie

Radish is a fantastic alkaline keto veggie that is very often overlooked. I always say there is no need to look for expensive and over-priced superfoods. Why not focus on what is already freely available? Radishes are very alkalizing and good for your liver and immune system. They are also very refreshing!

Servings: 1-2

Ingredients:

- Half cup radish, washed
- 1 small avocado, peeled and pitted
- A handful of fresh arugula leaves
- 1 cup full-fat coconut milk (no added sugar)
- Half cup of water
- Pinch of Himalaya salt to taste
- Pinch of black pepper to taste
- Optional: red chili pepper

Instructions:

1. Blend all the ingredients.
2. Serve in a smoothie glass or in a soup bowl- this smoothie can also be turned into a delicious soup.

If you serve this smoothie as a soup, feel free to add in some protein. It can be plant-based protein, for example, some nuts and seeds, or hard-boiled eggs. My husband loves to add in some smoked salmon or bacon.

Bonus – Mediterranean Smoothie Recipes

Cilantro Oriental Alkaline Keto Smoothie

Cilantro is a miraculous alkaline herb with potent antioxidant properties. While making a curry can be very time-consuming, why not enjoy cilantro in a simple smoothie that you can make in less than 5 minutes).

Servings: 2-3

Ingredients:

- 2 cups coconut or almond milk
- 2 tablespoons coconut oil
- A handful of fresh cilantro leaves
- 1 small red bell pepper, sliced and seeded
- 1 teaspoon curry powder
- Pinch of Himalaya salt to taste
- Pinch of black pepper powder to taste

Instructions:

1. Combine all the ingredients in a blender.
2. Process until smooth.
3. Taste to check if you need to add more salt or spices.
4. Pour into a smoothie glass or a small soup bowl and enjoy!

Vitamin C Alkaline Keto Power

This delicious smoothie is jam-packed with vitamin C coming from alkaline and keto friendly fruits like limes and lemons. Now, I understand that looking at the ingredients of this recipe, you may be feeling a bit "turned off." Yes, alkaline keto smoothies are very different to usual "sweet fruity smoothies."

But, give it a try. It tastes great! Very similar to natural, Greek yogurt. You can also use this smoothie recipe to season your salads. Most salad seasonings are full of crappy carbs, sugars and a ton of chemicals, while this smoothie is 100% natural! Another suggestion is - you could use this smoothie recipe to make a smoothie bowl by adding in some nuts and seeds. Once you have tried this smoothie, you will get my point for sure!

Servings: 2

Ingredients:

- 1 big avocado, peeled, pitted and sliced
- Half lemon, peeled and sliced
- 1 cup of coconut milk
- 1 teaspoon coconut oil
- Pinch of Himalaya salt
- Pinch of black pepper
- A few slices of lime to garnish

Instructions:

1. Place all the ingredients in a blender.
2. Process until smooth.
3. Serve in a smoothie glass and garnish with a few lime slices.
4. Drink to your health and enjoy!

Hormone Rebalancer Natural Energy Smoothie

This smoothie recipe is a fantastic option if you don't like green smoothies, but you still want to experience all the health benefits of alkaline keto smoothies.

This recipe uses stevia which is a natural sweetener, very often used both on keto and alkaline diets.

Although, let me remind you that once your taste buds have adapted, you will be able to do without any sweeteners easily.

Still, if you need one- go for stevia.

Servings: 1-2

Ingredients:

- 1 big grapefruit, peeled and halved
- 1 cup water (filtered, preferably alkaline)
- 1 inch of ginger, peeled
- 1 tablespoon coconut oil
- Half teaspoon maca powder
- Stevia to sweeten, if desired

Instructions:

1. Blend all the ingredients in a blender.
2. Serve and enjoy!

CONCLUSION

Don't forget to pick up your FREE GIFT...

Free Complimentary eBook

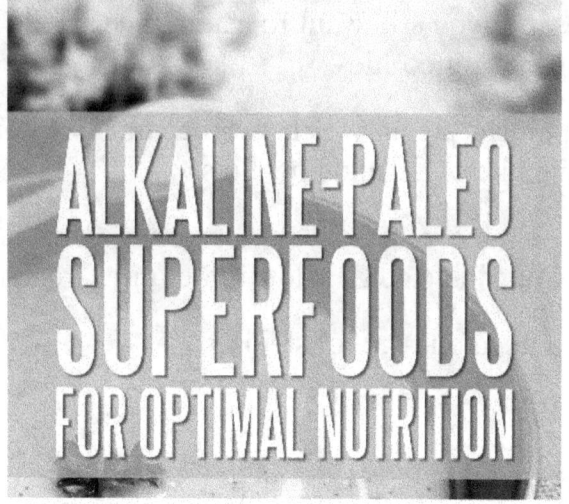

Sign up link:

www.yourwellnessbooks.com/newsletter

Problems with your download?

Contact us: elenajamesbooks@gmail.com

Conclusion

What's the key to success in healthy lifestyle and dieting?

I think it's all about <u>seeking balance</u>. The Mediterranean Diet provides us with a wonderful solution that is healthy, delicious, and of course, balanced.

Your homework is to prepare a shopping list and get started on cooking now.

I tried my best to present dishes that are quick and easy, as well as more traditional, family recipes. I also encourage you to use your imagination. If you want to be a good and healthy cook- simply keep practicing.

If you would like to learn more about healthy cooking and dieting please check out my other books.

I strongly recommend you familiarize yourself with the alkaline diet as well, and try to combine it with the Mediterranean style of eating. The benefits will be amazing!

You will also realize that it is very easy to get addicted to a healthy lifestyle.

Finally, if you enjoyed my book and it gave you some new cooking ideas I would really appreciate it if you could post your honest review-Help me spread the word and share your experiences with other readers.

I wish you vibrant health,

Elena Garcia

www.YourWellnessBooks.com

CONCLUSION
More books by Elena Garcia & Your Wellness Books

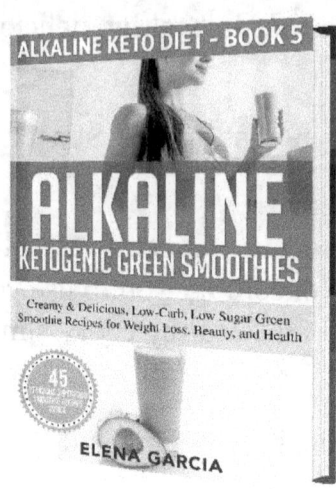
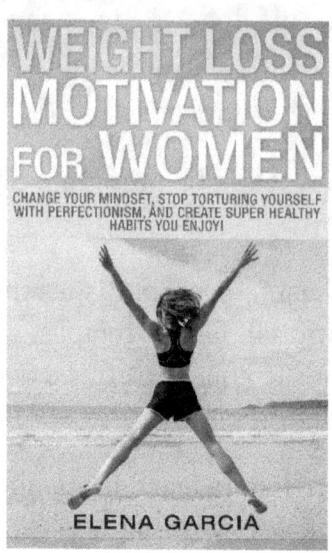

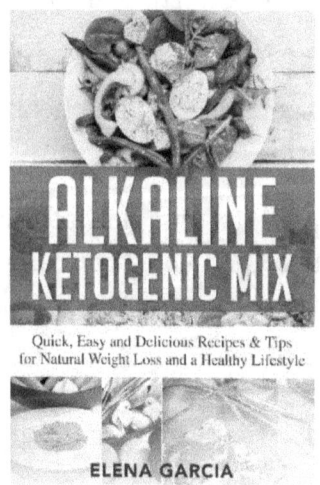
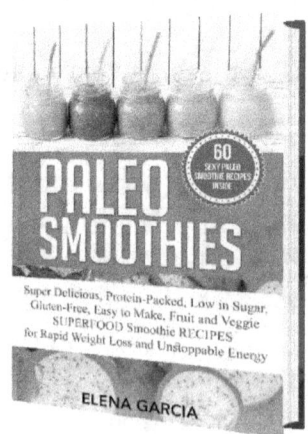

Available on Amazon and www.YourWellnessBooks.com/books

CONCLUSION

Recommended Resources Mentioned in This Book

1. Alkaline Acid Charts available at:

www.YourWellnessBooks.com/charts

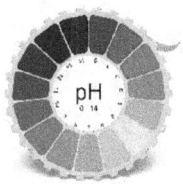

2. Alkaline Cleanse – discover how to lose weight and get rid of sugar cravings without feeling hungry or deprived:

www.YourWellnessBooks.com/cleanse

3. Sustainable weight loss after 40, 50, 60, and even 70…

www.YourWellnessBooks.com/weight-loss

CONCLUSION

www.ingramcontent.com/pod-product-compliance
Lightning Source LLC
Chambersburg PA
CBHW071524080526
44588CB00011B/1554